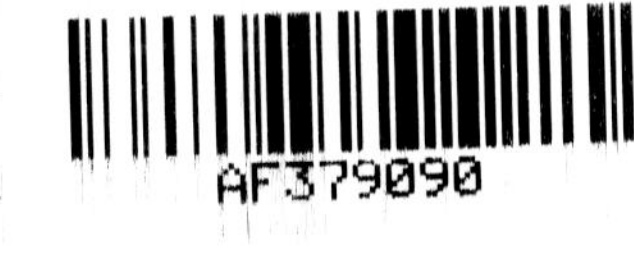

Made in the USA
Monee, IL
07 July 2026

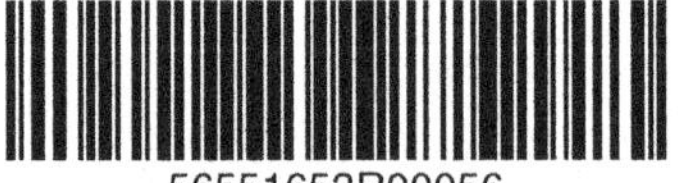

56551653R00056